Lessons from a Hospital Bed

LESSONS

FROM A

HOSPITAL

BED

John Piper

Foreword by
Joni Eareckson Tada

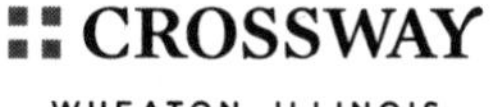

WHEATON, ILLINOIS

Lessons from a Hospital Bed

Published by Crossway
1300 Crescent Street
Wheaton, Illinois 60187

Cover design: Jeff Miller, Faceout Studio

Cover image: Shutterstock.com

First printing 2016

Printed in the United States of America

All emphases in Scripture quotations have been added by the author.

Trade paperback ISBN: 978-1-4335-5043-0
ePub ISBN: 978-1-4335-5046-1
PDF ISBN: 978-1-4335-5044-7
Mobipocket ISBN: 978-1-4335-5045-4

Library of Congress Cataloging-in-Publication Data

Names: Piper, John, 1946–
Title: Lessons from a hospital bed / John Piper ; foreword by Joni Eareckson Tada.
Description: Wheaton : Crossway, 2016. | Includes index.
Identifiers: LCCN 2015019155 (print) | LCCN 2015037842 (ebook) | ISBN 9781433550430 (tp) | ISBN 9781433550447 (pdf) | ISBN 9781433550454 (mobi) | ISBN 9781433550461 (epub)
Subjects: LCSH: Hospital patients—Religious life. | Patients—Religious life. | Diseases—Religious aspects—Christianity.
Classification: LCC BV4910.P56 2016 (print) | LCC BV4910 (ebook) | DDC 248.8/6—dc23
LC record available at http://lccn.loc.gov/2015019155

Crossway is a publishing ministry of Good News Publishers.

DP 25 24 23 22 21 20 19 18 17 16
14 13 12 11 10 9 8 7 6 5 4 3 2 1

Contents

Foreword:
Before You Begin . . .

I know hospitals. I wish I didn't, but over the years I've become all too acquainted with their stale corridors and freezing-cold operating rooms. It started back in 1967 when a reckless dive into shallow water snapped my neck, leaving me a quadriplegic. When they rushed me to the hospital on that hot July afternoon, I had no idea I wouldn't be discharged until April 1969.

One morning I was lying on a gurney in the hallway outside the urology clinic. After two hours of waiting and counting ceiling tiles, a lab worker came through the doors to announce I would be "first after lunch break." I moaned. My shoulders were already hurting from lying flat so long. As the urology staff headed to the cafeteria, my heart sank. More to the point, I nearly choked in a flood of fear and claustrophobia.

Crying was out. There was no one around to wipe my tears. So I decided to comfort my soul with a hymn. In no more than a whisper, I sang a favorite from church choir:

> Be still, my soul: the Lord is on thy side.
> Bear patiently the cross of grief or pain.
> Leave to thy God to order and provide;
> In every change he faithful will remain.
> Be still, my soul: thy best, thy heavenly
> Friend
> Through thorny ways leads to a joyful
> end!

I was only seventeen years old, or maybe eighteen, but that moment defined how I would engage life in a hospital. My stay would *not* be a jail sentence. Come hell or high water, I determined that this hospital would be, well, a gymnasium for my soul, a proving ground for my faith, and a mission field for God.

Sound improbable for a teenager? It is. And looking back, it was. Yet I was enough of a Christ follower to know I *had* to hold onto biblical hope, or else I would go crazy. Yes, I was still wrestling against depression, still struggling with how to actually *live* without the use of my hands or legs—even after I was released from the hospital in 1969. But I would *not* allow myself to sink into despair. That small, resolute act made all the difference, not only then but also years later when I battled stage 3 cancer and chronic pain.

This is why I love the little book you are holding in your hands. You may think its chapters are too short to carry any real weight, but they are perfectly pithy: wisdom delivered through a peashooter. In *Lessons from a Hospital Bed,* John Piper does not have to vet himself as a seasoned navigator of hospitals (much like good ob-gyns never have to give birth to a baby). His credentials come from his Spirit-breathed ability to tell you what's prudent—what the *right* thing to do is with all the hours you'll log while languishing in your hospital bed.

So please, don't plow through this booklet too quickly. Read its lessons prayerfully and act on their counsel intentionally. Next to your Bible, this little book is your best guide in making certain your hospital stay does genuine good for your soul.

As John has often said, "Don't waste your suffering." And friend, I trust his *Lessons from a Hospital Bed* will help you avoid doing just that during your time in the hospital. It's not a jail—it's a gymnasium. So flip the page and get started. And may God's healing hand of grace rest on you during your illness.

Joni Eareckson Tada
Joni and Friends International
 Disability Center
Fall 2015

The Setting

I wrote this little book in two stages. The heart of it came soon after I was hospitalized for thirty hours due to an unexplained blood clot in my lung. The lessons were fresh from that experience. The rest of it was added about a year later as I reflected more on what God has taught me over the years through sickness and suffering.

I do not write as a veteran sufferer. My life has been too easy for that claim. I assume that most of you are going through more than I ever have. I have stayed overnight in the hospital only three times (not counting when I was born!)—twice relating to prostate cancer, once for the blood clot. Compared to what some of you have been through, that is very minor.

People ask me, "How's your health?" I used to answer, "Fine." I don't answer that way anymore. I say, "I feel fine." There's a difference. The day before I went for my annual prostate exam, I felt fine. The day after, I was told I had cancer. In other words, I was not fine. So even as I write these words, I do not know if I am fine. For all I know, I have cancer right now. Or perhaps some blood clot is ready to break off and go to my lung.

I mention these things to simply say this: you and I are both very vulnerable right now. You may be in the hospital and I at home. But neither of us knows for sure how well or how sick we are. So instead of saying, "I'm fine," we say, "I feel fine." This fits with what the Bible tell us:

> Come now, you who say, "Today or tomorrow we will go into such and such a town and spend a year there and trade and make a profit"—yet you do not know what tomorrow will bring. What is your life? For you are a mist that appears for a little time and then vanishes.

> Instead you ought to say, "If the Lord wills, we will live and do this or that." (James 4:13–15)

If the Lord wills, we will live. So we are not as vulnerable as it seems. Our lives are in the mighty hands of God. If he wills, we live. We are immortal until his purpose for us is done. No adversary, no disease can take us out if God wills for us to live. Nothing could be more secure than to be held in the saving hands of God.

But now I have started quoting the Bible. Maybe you didn't expect that. Or maybe you did. If I were you, I would want to know why John Piper quotes the Bible. Where is this writer coming from? So it seems good to me that I should begin by telling you what I believe.

I hope this confession accomplishes two things. One is candor. I want to be completely honest and open about what I believe and where I'm getting my thoughts. The other is encouragement. I am a Christian because I believe these things are true and are the best news in the world, especially in the hospital. In other words, I want to be honest and encouraging.

I know you don't have time or strength to read a long treatise. So I'll tell you where I am coming from in ten short summaries (part 1). If you want, you can just skip these and go straight to part 2, the lessons I learned in the hospital.

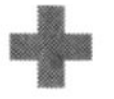

Part 1

TEN BELIEFS I BROUGHT TO THE HOSPITAL

All of us have beliefs about life and death, about good and evil, and about God. If someone is going to presume to give you counsel about your time in the hospital, it seems good that you should know what he believes and why. So here are ten things I believe. I took these into the hospital with me when I was sick. I banked on them while I was there. And I brought them out again, more sure than ever that they are true.

1

The Bible is the Word of God and should be trusted.

John Piper's opinion about your suffering has no authority. God's Word does. If you ask me, "But how do you know the Bible is the Word of God?" my short answer would be, "There is a glory that shines through it, which fits perfectly with the God-shaped template in your heart." When your mind is clearest, you know the voice of God. As Jesus says, "My sheep hear my voice, and I know them, and they follow me" (John 10:27).

Deep down you know God. That's what the Bible says: "What can be known about God is plain to them, because God has shown it to them" (Rom. 1:19). Just as God's world makes clear that he is its Maker (Ps. 19:1), so God's Word makes clear that he is its Author.

It's similar to the way you know that honey is honey. Scientists may say this jar contains honey because of chemical experiments. But *you* know it's honey because you tasted it. Similarly, there is a divine sweetness in God's Word. It touches a part of you that you know was put there by God. Thus the psalmist exclaims, "How sweet are your words to my taste, sweeter than honey to my mouth!" (Ps. 119:103).

So when Jesus says, "Scripture cannot be broken" (John 10:35), and when Saint Paul says, "All Scripture is breathed out by God" (2 Tim. 3:16), and when Saint Peter says, the authors of Scripture "were carried along by the Holy Spirit" (2 Pet. 1:21), your heart says, *yes*.

You have tasted. You have seen. And there is a sweet, deep assurance that these words are true. Your whole soul resonates with statements like these: "The sum of your word is truth" (Ps. 119:160); "Forever, O Lord, your word is firmly fixed in the heavens" (Ps. 119:89); "Every word of God proves true" (Prov. 30:5).

When this happens, the whole truth of God washes over you in the hospital with incomparable comfort: "When the cares of my heart are many, your consolations cheer my soul" (Ps. 94:19); "The LORD is near to the brokenhearted and saves the crushed in spirit. Many are the afflictions of the righteous, but the LORD delivers him out of them all" (Ps. 34:18–19).

No man can comfort your soul the way God can. His comfort is unshakable. It comes from his Word, the Bible. That is my first belief. And all the others are based on this one.

2

God is good.

The Bible tells us, "The Lord is good, a stronghold in the day of trouble; he knows those who take refuge in him" (Nah. 1:7). "God is light, and in him is no darkness at all" (1 John 1:5). "For the Lord is good; his steadfast love endures forever, and his faithfulness to all generations" (Ps. 100:5).

But in the hospital, we are surrounded by suffering. There is no place quite like it. In the outside world, pain seems to dissolve in the water of ordinary life. But in the hospital, it's as if the water has been boiled away, leaving only the concentrated sediment of suffering. You can see it and smell it and hear it.

You may be tempted to ask, *Is God good?* There is so much suffering in the world that he made! Let George Mueller give God's answer from the Bible. Mueller is famous for building orphanages for destitute children in England in the nineteenth century. In 1870, when he was sixty-five, his wife of forty years died. He loved her deeply. He spoke at her funeral and chose Psalm 119:68 as his text: "You are good and do good." He recalled in the sermon how he held on to this truth:

> All will be according to His own blessed character. Nothing but that, which is good, like Himself, can proceed from Him. If he pleases to take my dearest wife, it will be good, like Himself. What I have to do, as His child, is to be satisfied with what my Father does, that I may glorify Him. After this my soul not only aimed, but this, my soul, by God's grace, attained to. I was satisfied with God.*

Even when we are surrounded by suffering in the hospital, God is still good.

* George Mueller, *A Narrative of Some of the Lord's Dealings with George Müller, Written by Himself, Jehovah Magnified. Addresses by George Müller Complete and Unabridged* (Muskegon, MI: Dust and Ashes, 2003), 2:398–99.

3

God is wise and knows everything.

God knows absolutely everything about your body and its disease. Compared to his knowledge of the universe, all the scientists and all the libraries in the world are like children and first-grade readers. There is nothing he does not know and understand perfectly:

> Oh, the depth of the riches and wisdom and knowledge of God! How unsearchable are his judgments and how inscrutable his ways! (Rom. 11:33)

> The LORD is the everlasting God,
> the Creator of the ends of the earth.
> . . . his understanding is
> unsearchable. (Isa. 40:28)

And with this infinite knowledge, he is infinitely wise. He uses his infinite knowledge to accomplish all his wise purposes:

> With God are wisdom and might;
> he has counsel and understanding.
> (Job 12:13)

> O Lord, how manifold are your works!
> In wisdom have you made them all.
> (Ps. 104:24)

> Blessed be the name of God forever and ever,
> to whom belong wisdom and might.
> (Dan. 2:20)

God means for this to comfort us in our trouble. We know this because he tells us to pray for our needs but not to use a lot of words, as if he were reluctant: "Do not heap up empty phrases as the Gentiles do . . . for your Father knows what you need before you ask him" (Matt. 6:7–8). He knows what you need. Don't be anxious about your daily needs; "your heavenly Father knows that you need them all" (Matt. 6:32). He knows.

And in his wisdom, every need will be met: "My God will supply every need of yours according to his riches in glory in Christ Jesus" (Phil. 4:19). And so we proclaim, "To the only wise God be glory forevermore through Jesus Christ! Amen" (Rom. 16:27).

4

God is totally in control.

Some find this comforting. Some find it incredible. Some find it blasphemous. Some find it cruel. I am in that first group. It is a great comfort to me that whatever happens to me, and to those I love, is not in the control of meaningless chance or malevolent demons. God is good, and God is wise; so it is good news that God is in control.

God says, "My counsel shall stand, and I will accomplish all my purpose" (Isa. 46:10), and, "I am the LORD. . . . Is anything too hard for me?" (Jer. 32:27). And we respond with Job, "I know that you can do all things, and that no purpose of yours can be thwarted" (Job 42:2). And with Christ we say, "With God all things are possible" (Matt. 19:26).

Why is it good news to say, with Jesus, that not a single sparrow falls to the ground apart from the will of our Father? Jesus tells us why: "You are of more value than many sparrows" (Matt. 10:31).

When we are sick or dying, we may not see the kindness of God as easily as when we were well. But that is why we need God's Word. Experience is not a reliable guide. God is.

When sickness and Satan and maybe even other people threaten our lives, we need to hear God say to us what he said to Joseph's brothers. They had sold Joseph into slavery (Gen. 37:28), and now he was their master in Egypt. But here is what he said: "As for you, you meant evil against me, but God meant it for good" (Gen. 50:20).

Not just "God *used* it for good" but "God *meant* it for good." They had an evil purpose. God had a good one. This is the key to all comfort in suffering. However evil Satan's aims are in our lives, God's aims are good. This is a huge comfort when everything else looks bleak.

5

Sin is the ugly origin of ugly disease.

I don't mean your sickness is a specific punishment for your sin. I mean all sickness is owing to the sin of the first man and woman, Adam and Eve. Sickness and suffering come to the most godly people in the world. All our trials are God's merciful refining of our faith as gold (1 Pet. 1:6–7). But there is no simple correlation between specific sins and specific sufferings.

When our first parents rebelled against God and took matters into their own hands, God turned the whole world into a painful parable of the ugliness of that act. The Bible says that God "subjected [creation] to futility" and gave it over to the "bondage [of] corruption" (Rom. 8:20–21). As we lie in the hospital and listen to the sound of pain, what we should be hearing is, *Sin is ugly*.

6

Jesus Christ died and rose to save sinners.

The most comforting news we can possibly hear in the hospital, or anywhere, is that God shows his love for those who have rebelled against him. He has sent his Son, Jesus Christ, to bear the punishment that sinners deserve.

It is a horrible thing to lie in a hospital bed and wonder if we are dying and yet have no peace with God. But it is a wonderful thing to be able to lie there and know that even if we die, we will not be condemned but have eternal life.

God made that kind of peace possible. The link between our guilty souls and God's love is faith in Christ. What did he do?

- "He himself bore our sins in his body on the tree" (1 Pet. 2:24).
- "Christ also suffered once for sins, the righteous for the unrighteous, that he might bring us to God" (1 Pet. 3:18).
- God "made him to be sin who knew no sin, so that in him we might become the righteousness of God" (2 Cor. 5:21).
- "God shows his love for us in that while we were still sinners, Christ died for us" (Rom. 5:8).
- "God so loved the world, that he gave his only Son, that whoever believes in him should not perish but have eternal life" (John 3:16).

When we trust in this amazing work of Christ, we can rest in the promise of Romans 8:1: "There is therefore now no condemnation for those who are in Christ Jesus." Is anything sweeter than to fall asleep, even in a hospital bed, knowing that whether we live or die, God is for us?

When I was given my cancer diagnosis, this is what the Lord gave me: Live or die, you are mine.

For God has not destined us for wrath, but to obtain salvation through our Lord Jesus Christ, who died for us so that whether we are awake or asleep we might live with him. (1 Thess. 5:9–10)

7

Sickness is not God's first design or final plan for this world.

Sickness is not the way it was supposed to be. When God created the world, he "saw everything that he had made, and behold, it was very good" (Gen. 1:31). There was no sickness before sin. And the day is coming when sickness will be no more. God's purpose is to rid the world entirely of sin and unrighteousness and suffering. He will make the whole world new:

> He will wipe away every tear from their eyes, and death shall be no more, neither shall there be mourning, nor crying, nor pain anymore, for the former things have passed away. (Rev. 21:4)

No more hospitals. No more chemotherapy. No more wheelchairs or crutches or braces. No more antibiotics or morphine. No more surgeries or physical therapies. In one all-encompassing healing for his redeemed world, God will put things right. For this we wait eagerly—and even groan: "We ourselves, who have the firstfruits of the Spirit, groan inwardly as we wait eagerly for adoption as sons, the redemption of our bodies" (Rom. 8:23).

8

Satan is real and cruel but not in control.

Satan is God's first and greatest enemy. But he is not God's equal. God could at any moment put him totally out of commission. Evidently, God thinks it best, for now, to let Satan tempt and, at times, torment—and even kill—his people (Rev. 2:10).

This is the story of Job. Satan had to get God's permission to make him sick (Job 2:4–7). Similarly, he had to get God's permission to tempt Peter (Luke 22:31–32). Satan is not free to do anything he pleases. He does, the Bible says, go around like a lion, trying to destroy the faith of God's people—including those in hospital beds (1 Pet. 5:8–9). But he is on a leash. He cannot reach you unless God lets him.

God has given us the shield of faith to quench Satan's fiery darts (Eph. 6:16). And he has promised to deliver us from Satan's jaws: "Submit yourselves therefore to God. Resist the devil, and he will flee from you" (James 4:7).

And what a sweet and strong promise for those of you who are suffering right now:

> Resist [the devil], firm in your faith, knowing that the same kinds of suffering are being experienced by your brotherhood throughout the world. And after you have suffered a little while, the God of all grace, who has called you to his eternal glory in Christ, will himself restore, confirm, strengthen, and establish you. To him be the dominion forever and ever. Amen. (1 Pet. 5:9–11)

9

Healing is possible now and certain later.

God still heals. Sometimes he heals miraculously. Sometimes he heals through the medical means put in the hands of doctors. God does not promise to heal all sickness in this age. When the Bible says, "By his wounds you have been healed" (1 Pet. 2:24), it does not specify when.

Paul makes plain that one effect of humanity's fall into sin is that even Christians "groan inwardly as we wait eagerly for adoption as sons, the redemption of our bodies" (Rom. 8:23). That means we must wait till the second coming. Until then, Christians will groan because of disease and calamity.

But even though our final inheritance includes the total healing of all God's children (Rev. 21:4), there are early disbursements of the inheritance to be enjoyed now. One way to look at it is to say that the kingdom of God has come—in part.

Jesus said, "If it is by the finger of God that I cast out demons, then the kingdom of God has come upon you" (Luke 11:20). And again, "The kingdom of God is in the midst of you" (Luke 17:21). And the coming of the kingdom includes healing from the king. Jesus sent the apostles out "to proclaim the kingdom of God and to heal" (Luke 9:2). So if the kingdom is here in measure, healing is here in measure too.

So James told all the churches of his day, "Is anyone among you sick? Let him call for the elders of the church, and let them pray over him. . . . Therefore, confess your sins to one another and pray for one another, that you may be healed" (James 5:14, 16). Don't be ashamed to ask for such prayer. And trust the outcome to your Father who knows what is best.

10

Your life and your illness are not meaningless.

You are not the victim of random cell mutations or accidental genetic anomalies or rogue viruses or maverick molecules or chance misfortunes. If that is the kind of world we live in, I would certainly not be writing this short book. There would be no meaning and no hope. You and I would be no more significant than the mattress you lie on—just a more complicated combination of molecules.

Events have *meaning* when there is someone in charge who *means*. And there is. God speaks over your life these words: "My counsel shall stand, and I will accomplish all my purpose" (Isa. 46:10). He is busy at this very moment working all things together for your everlasting good (Rom. 8:28). He cannot fail: "The counsel of the Lord stands forever, the plans of his heart to all generations" (Ps. 33:11).

Doctors and nurses and family members all have plans for you. But one plan is sure. One plan gives unshakable and eternal meaning to your life. "Many are the plans in the mind of a man," the ancient sage observes, "but it is the purpose of the Lord that will stand" (Prov. 19:21).

You need not worry about the slightest slipup. Not a bird falls to the ground apart from your heavenly Father's will (Matt. 10:29). Every throw of the dice in every casino, not to mention every medical procedure, is guided by God for God's purposes: "The lot is cast into the lap [the therapy is chosen], but its every decision is from the Lord" (Prov. 16:33).

For a season, God has made you like a helpless little child. Trust him. He is a good

Father. All-wise, all-strong, all-loving. Rest in him. He has much to teach you. This is what I found when my time came. And what I hope I will find again. For there will almost certainly be an "again."

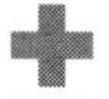

Part 2

TEN LESSONS FROM MY HOSPITAL BED

Some of these lessons took me off guard. I was not expecting some of the battles I had to fight. In all of them, I needed God's help. I was surprised how difficult it was for me to focus on anything and, therefore, how spiritually vulnerable I felt.

I'm used to focusing my mind on God's truth—especially on his promises—and fighting off the temptations of fear and anger. But when focus is hard, trust is hard. So don't assume as you read these lessons that they came easy for me. They didn't.

Not wanting to waste this experience, I jotted down the lessons that were most immediate and most pressing. It was good for me. Maybe if I list some of them, you will be helped when your time comes. That's my prayer.

1

Don't murmur about delays and inefficiencies in the hospital when you are getting medical care that surpasses by a hundredfold what is available in 90 percent of the world.

Instead of focusing on the fact that your nurse isn't responding or the man in the next bed is snoring or the intravenous device is beeping or the ice chips have run out, think about the fact that 150 years ago you would probably be dead by this point. And if not, you might be groaning in unrelieved pain with no morphine to help. And you may have no clue what's wrong with you or whether or not you are dying.

We modern Americans do not suffer well. We expect things to work. We expect help when we feel we need it. We expect relief from a pill. We expect those who serve us to be courteous and respectful. And we do not expect to be told there is nothing that can be done.

So we are prone to complain. I certainly am. And I am ashamed of it. It contradicts all that I believe about God. It makes him look weak or foolish or inattentive or uncaring or helpless. He is none of these. And so my complaining tells lies about him. And I am sorry.

It is amazing what the Bible says about grumbling:

> Do all things without grumbling or disputing, that you may be blameless and innocent, children of God without blemish in the midst of a crooked and twisted generation, among whom you shine as lights in the world. (Phil. 2:14–15)

Do you want to "shine as a light" in the medical world? The Bible says, the brightness of your shining is the absence of your grumbling. Amazing!

Why is freedom from grumbling so bright and amazing? Because grumbling is the most natural thing in the world. When we grumble, we act like everybody else. You don't need the Holy Spirit to grumble. You don't need Christ to grumble. You don't need love to grumble. And you don't need faith to grumble. All you need is your own entitled self.

So here was my first lesson. I needed to look to Christ. Here was my example and my helper: "Christ also suffered for you, leaving you an example, so that you might follow in his steps. . . . When he was reviled, he did not revile in return; when he suffered, he did not threaten, but continued entrusting himself to him who judges justly" (1 Pet. 2:21, 23).

We are in the hospital by design, on a mission. Let your light shine.

2

Don't let yourself be spiritually numbed by the ceaseless barrage of sounds, noises, television, and chatter that surrounds you in the hospital.

I was amazed at the ceaselessness of sound. Maybe it's different for others. But for me, there was almost no letup. Not even in the middle of the night. The nurses were chattering. The helpers who came to serve my roommate at 3:00 a.m. conversed like it was midafternoon. Televisions blared continuously. A strange beeping or buzzing or humming was almost constant. I longed for silence.

This was a trial to my spirit. In the very

moment when I needed to be still and know that God is God, my heart was off balance with distraction. This was a surprise to me. It took me off guard. I had to pray and concentrate and recite Scripture to myself to regain my spiritual stability. "Oh, guard my soul, and deliver me!" (Ps. 25:20).

Perhaps, if you find yourself in the same condition, a few passages from God's Word will help you enjoy God's peace in the midst of noise:

- "You keep him in perfect peace whose mind is stayed on you, because he trusts in you" (Isa. 26:3).
- "Thus said the Lord GOD, the Holy One of Israel, 'In returning and rest you shall be saved; in quietness and in trust shall be your strength'" (Isa. 30:15).
- "In peace I will both lie down and sleep; for you alone, O LORD, make me dwell in safety" (Ps. 4:8).
- "Do not be anxious about anything, but in everything by prayer and supplication with thanksgiving let your requests be

made known to God. And the peace of God, which surpasses all understanding, will guard your hearts and your minds in Christ Jesus" (Phil. 4:6–7).

- "May the God of hope fill you with all joy and peace in believing, so that by the power of the Holy Spirit you may abound in hope" (Rom. 15:13).

Amid all the sounds and smells and interruptions and goings and comings—not to mention the discomfort and pain and fear—may the God of peace quiet your soul and give you sweet fellowship with Jesus.

3

Don't default to the television.

The hospital makes this the easiest thing for you to do. Many hospitals provide a television for every bed. It's as close as the button by your head. I don't have a television at home, and the reason for that choice, and for this advice, is not the boogeymen of sex and violence (which are real). It's the more subtle and pervasive dehumanizing banality of most television programming. This is the last thing a person needs who knows he is standing on the brink of eternity.

When I listened to what the patient next to me was watching on television, what appalled me was not the sensuality (which was bad enough) but the emptiness of it all—the triviality, the silliness, the juvenile hollowness. Grown people were all acting as if life was vaudeville. I was embarrassed for them. Not because they had lost their clothes but because they had lost their glorious humanity—not to mention any sense of Godwardness.

And all this was in stark contrast to the horrific condition of the man next to me. He was miserable. And seriously ill. The juxtaposition of the triviality of television and the majesty of a suffering being created in the image of God was tragic. You would never guess from television that the human soul possesses a magnificence and greatness and wonder, especially in how it relates to the Creator of the world.

Don't default to the television. Give yourself to reading, listening to, or thinking about things that ennoble your soul and that put it in touch with the glory that it is and the Glory it was made for. Perhaps before you go into the hospital, if it's not a sudden event, prepare a playlist of worship music and Christ-centered messages on your mobile device. Or if that is a foreign idea to you, ask someone to help you so that you can put your earphones in and do as much good for your soul as the doctors are doing for your body.

As the apostle Paul exhorts us, "If then you have been raised with Christ, seek the things that are above, where Christ is, seated at the right hand of God. Set your minds on things that are above, not on things that are on earth" (Col. 3:1–2).

4

Pray for the patients near you, and if possible—without undue offense—see if your roommates will let you pray for them and give them words of hope in Jesus.

I was not satisfied with my attempt at doing this with the poor man next to me. He was so miserable. But I did try. And before I left, I wrote him a note in a book about Jesus and left it with him, asking the Lord to bless him. I did the same for the nurse who served me so generously with a smile.

You are nowhere by mere coincidence. My wife likes to use the term "God-incidence." That's right. These are all divine appointments. You have no idea what the simplest witness to Christ may bring.

During my many years of pastoral ministry, we would listen to the testimonies of people who were joining the church. They would tell us the story of how God brought them to himself. More often than not, the story included multiple encounters with Christians and with the gospel. In other words, rarely did people say they trusted Christ the first time they heard about him. Or the second. Or the third. But at some point, God opened their eyes, and they saw the truth and beauty of Jesus.

What that means is that none of our efforts to speak the good news of Christ is wasted. It may or may not lead immediately to someone's conversion. But we never know what God may do with those words.

For example, I was a water-safety instructor and camp counselor in the summer of 1967 at a Christian camp. I also had five guys in my cabin whom I was supposed to point to Christ. None of them seemed to me to be real

Christians. So I did my best each night to say something winsome and true about Christ. They did not seem very interested.

I had to leave camp before the final evening. Later I was told that several of those guys made professions of faith at the closing event.

Don't ever think you are wasting your words when you speak for Jesus. You are in this hospital at this time in this room for a reason. Surely we can apply Jesus's words from the Gospel of Luke in this way:

> You will be brought before kings and governors [and doctors and nurses and patients] for my name's sake. This will be your opportunity to bear witness. (Luke 21:12–13)

5

Realize that physical pain makes focusing on God's promises more difficult and demands greater concentrating effort.

It's not just the barrage of sounds that disorient our souls; it's the pain. I don't want this to blindside you. The very thing we need God for can blur our vision of God.

At this point, it is so important that you have in your heart some very simple, short biblical truths about God that you can declare to yourself. Long complex reasoning about God's sovereignty and goodness won't work in this situation, because the pain is too disorienting. It doesn't allow the mind to work at full capacity.

What you need is this: "The Lord is my Shepherd." Period. "Christ gave himself for me." Period. "I will never leave you." Period. "Nothing is too hard for the Lord." Period. "Everything works for good." Period. These are like white stones with your name on them. And you hold them in your hand as you groan and wait.

So while you have the mental capacity and freedom from pain to do it, read your Bible with an eye searching for these kinds of treasures. It's as if you were a son being sent off to war by his dad. At the last minute, the dad puts a tiny metal football in his son's hand. The son clasps it firmly and knows what it means: "We had great times together, and I love you."

My dad did that for me. I was about to get on the airplane in New York to go to Germany to study. He was not able to be there. He reached me from a phone booth near Radio City Music Hall. The last thing he said was,

"Fear not, for I am with you; be not dismayed, for I am your God; I will strengthen you, I will help you, I will uphold you with my righteous right hand." It was Isaiah 41:10 spoken directly to me, his son. I probably quoted it to myself a thousand times during the years I was away.

Over the years, when I have visited people in the hospital, especially those about to enter serious surgery, I have tried to give them very short and glorious truths that they would be able to remember as the anesthesia put them under. Just a few words. My suggestion is that you grasp on to one of these. Pain disorients the mind. But one small word of truth can keep you focused. Here's the one I used during my cancer surgery: "You are not destined for wrath!" (see 1 Thess. 5:9).

6

Reach out to a friend or family member to help you.

Often the suddenness of a hospitalization leaves the patient disoriented and unable to think clearly about all the aspects of what's going on. This was certainly true for me. Questions needed to be asked, and my mind was not at full strength.

I needed an advocate. My wife was there and was full of good questions for the doctors—about medications and lifestyle and diet and travel implications. As helpful as doctors are, they cannot think of all the things we might need to know in order to understand what has happened to us and in order to live wisely in the days to come. They need us to ask questions, and we need help to ask all the right questions.

Of course, not everyone has a wife or a husband to be there with them. So don't be afraid to ask for help. Find out when the doctor is going to come in and brief you, and ask your friend to be there. Give your friend permission to ask everything that comes to mind.

Asking for help like this is not easy to do. Most of us are used to being self-sufficient. Most of us don't like to feel helpless. Some people I have known over the years don't even tell others they are going to the hospital. They don't want to inconvenience anyone. This is not good. It overlooks an utterly crucial teaching from the Bible about who we are as Christians. We are parts of one body:

> The eye cannot say to the hand, "I have no need of you," nor again the head to the feet, "I have no need of you." On the contrary, the parts of the body that seem to be weaker are indispensable. (1 Cor. 12:21–22)

So be careful that you don't cloak the pride of self-sufficiency with the humility of unworthiness. It is more humble to reach out for help than to think we are serving others by not bothering them. Remember, "we are members one of another" (Eph. 4:25).

7

Accept the humiliation of wearing the same unflattering gown everyone else wears.

This is good for all of us. Most of the time we have control over our outward persona. We can dress in a way that presents us as more dignified (or self-sufficient) than we really are.

Picture the difference between the John Piper with his sports jacket preaching to thousands and the John Piper with his blue and white, split-down-the-back hospital robe hobbling to the bathroom in his non-slip, brown footies, dragging the intravenous roller with him.

This is a great reality check. We are all

weak, vulnerable, and fairly homely physical specimens who are getting less attractive all the time. But thanks be to God, "Though our outer self is wasting away, our inner self is being renewed day by day" (2 Cor. 4:16).

It is a wonderful thing, for example, to visit a dignified, mature, attractive Christian woman in the hospital and find her at peace, contented, and outgoing, even though her hair is not fixed, she has no makeup, and the gown is unflattering. This is wonderful because it reveals a deeper beauty. Her true beauty is in the fearless poise she has as a daughter of God. A sister of Christ. A soldier of the cross. An heir of the world.

So relax and don't be consumed with yourself and your appearance as people come into your life. Be more concerned with others than with yourself. Your identity and your value do not rise and fall with your looks. "You are of more value than many sparrows" (Luke 12:7).

8

Let the pain and misery of your body, and that of the people around you, remind you of the exceeding moral horror and spiritual ugliness of sin.

As I understand it, Romans 8:18–25 is Paul's commentary on humanity's fall into sin in Genesis 3. He is explaining the devastating physical effects on the creation caused by the moral evil that entered the world through Adam's sin. This means that God subjected the world to physical futility and misery to make a point about moral and spiritual reality.

Paul says, "The creation was subjected to futility" (Rom. 8:20). He refers to this "futility" as "bondage to corruption" (Rom. 8:21). The horrors and upheavals of disease and calamity are not ends in themselves; they are a "groaning together in the pains of childbirth" (Rom. 8:22). That is, they will usher in a new creation.

We all share in this groaning—a horrible groaning in the case of the worst cancers and maiming accidents: "We ourselves, [that is, we children of God,] who have the firstfruits of the Spirit, groan inwardly as we wait eagerly for adoption as sons, the redemption of our bodies" (Rom. 8:23). For God's children, this is not punishment. Christ bore that (Rom. 8:3). This is the lot of every human being—to bear the physical sign of the horrors of moral evil. This physical pain points to how ugly sin is.

If this sounds somewhat bleak for a hospital bed, consider this. Bleak thoughts about sin yield bright hope in God's grace. If we try to avoid hard things, we lose good things. Is that not why the Bible says, "It is better to go to the house of mourning than to go to the house of feasting, for this is the end of all mankind, and the living will lay it to heart" (Eccles. 7:2). As we lay it to heart, God teaches us wonderful things about himself and our future.

Let your groaning remind you of the disease and deformation you have been saved from—the ugliness of sin. Let it ignite a new passion in you to make war on the remnants of sin in your life.

9

Let the self-revelation of Jesus as the Great Physician be sweet to your soul, and preach to yourself that this light momentary affliction is working for you an eternal weight of glory.

Christ is all-sufficient for every situation. In the hospital, he is the preeminent Physician. Matthew 4:23 says he was able to heal "every disease and every affliction among the people." And at the last day, "he will wipe away every tear from their eyes, and death shall be no more, neither shall there be mourning, nor crying, nor pain anymore" (Rev. 21:4).

We should ask him, without hesitation, for healing and for relief from pain. We should trust him with the timing of his answer. But mainly we should realize with joy that, beyond all doubt, he has healed the deepest disease of everyone who trusts him—the damning disease of sin. As Jesus himself said, "Those who are well have no need of a physician, but those who are sick. I have not come to call the righteous but sinners to repentance" (Luke 5:31–32).

If God answers your prayer for healing with "Not yet," be assured of this: the affliction is not wasted. It is doing a kind of healing that will last for eternity. Here is an amazing promise:

> We do not lose heart. Though our outer self is wasting away, our inner self is being renewed day by day. For this light momentary affliction is preparing for us an eternal weight of glory beyond all comparison, as we look not to the things that are seen but to the things that are unseen. For the things that are seen are

> transient, but the things that are unseen are eternal. (2 Cor. 4:16–18)

This affliction is "preparing" a weight of glory. It really is. In other words, your suffering actually has an effect on your future glory. It is not just an obstacle to overcome. If we bear it in faith for the honor of Christ, it is a catapult to greater glory. Jesus is with you. Not even the worst pain is wasted in his hands.

10

Pray that none of these hospital hours, none of this pain, none of these fears, none of these relationships, none of this life-altering season will be wasted.

Satan wants to make your experience in the hospital meaningless and empty and fearful and trivial. Don't let him win this victory.

Pray. Pray as you go to the hospital. Pray in admissions. Pray on the gurney. Pray in the bed. Pray in the morning and in the middle of the night. Pray without ceasing.

You will probably be unable to formulate long, well-articulated prayers. The mind and body are too embattled. It is okay to pray with simple, short outbursts of need and thanks and praise:

- "Help me, Lord, to trust you."
- "Have mercy, Lord. I need you. I can hardly think."
- "Save me, Lord, from unbelief and sin."
- "I believe, Lord. Help my unbelief."
- "Thank you for your mercy."
- "Thank you, Jesus, that you loved me and gave yourself for me."
- "Thank you, Father, that there is no condemnation for me in Christ Jesus."
- "Use me, Jesus, to magnify your great worth."
- "Satisfy me in your steadfast love, no matter what happens here."

Remember how eager God is to hear you and help you. Yes, he is. He says so: "Fear not, little flock, for it is your Father's good pleasure to give you the kingdom" (Luke 12:32); "Call upon me in the day of trouble; I will deliver you, and you shall glorify me" (Ps. 50:15).

That will be the greatest result of your hospitalization: you will glorify him. Then you will know this has not been wasted.

Concluding Prayer

Father in heaven, in spite of all our uncertainties and all our embattled anxieties and all our discomfort, we say, great is the Lord and greatly to be praised. You are to be feared above all gods, for you made the heavens and the earth and our physical bodies. You sustain all things. You know all things. You rule all things. You are infinitely wise and powerful. And you are merciful—all-merciful—to all who receive your precious Son as the treasure of their lives.

So we do. We look to Christ. We look away from all self-reliance. Our trust is not finally in medicine or in man. We trust you. We call on you.

O God, hold fast to us. Preserve us by your

power. Sustain our faith. Don't let us waver in unbelief. Shine your irresistible light of glory into our hearts, and grant us to hope fully in your grace.

Don't let the pain be more than we can bear. Guard us from murmuring or complaining. Give us your peace that passes all human understanding. Keep our minds focused on your precious promises. And make us know your sweet presence at our bedside.

Grant your wisdom and skill, we pray, to the doctors and nurses. We thank you for the stunning advances in medical science that you have given to mankind. What a mercy to this undeserving world—including us!

And Father, we ask for your healing. You are the Great Physician. Nothing is too hard for you. To be with you in heaven would be our great pleasure. If that is your will, we embrace it with joyful hope. But there is work to do. There is family to care for. There are souls to touch and a church to serve and a world to win—and the second coming of your Son to hope in. So we ask to be raised up for your great glory.

Father, thank you for sending Jesus Christ to die for our sins. Thank you that "for our sake [you] made him to be sin who knew no sin, so that in him we might become the righteousness of God" (2 Cor. 5:21). O the wonder and privilege and peace of hearing you say to us, in Christ, "No condemnation. I do not appoint you for wrath" (see Rom. 8:1; 1 Thess. 5:9).

Into your hands we commit our bodies and our souls. In Jesus's name. Amen.

Scripture Index

My Rose Marie,

I read this book right after Ron died and it helped me through those first few weeks. So, I wanted to share it with you. I love you and am so very blessed to have you as my dearest friend and sister in Christ! Love,

Gail